I0790472

STEPS TO HEALTH

WALKING FOR FUN, FITNESS AND WELL-BEING

NANCY DURSO, MD

Contents

Introduction

What is more straightforward than walking? Most of us walk. It gets us from here to there. Why would I want to walk more than necessary? My husband always tries to get the closest parking spot to the store. I don't mind walking a little further. Walking is natural. It takes a minimal amount of equipment. You can do it by yourself or in a group. Most of us take walking for granted.

For several reasons, walking has always been the best form of exercise for me. In 2001, I tripped and broke my foot - a Lisfranc fracture across the middle of my right foot. After I was evaluated in the emergency room, an Orthopedic Surgeon was assigned to my case. He told me, "This is a bad break. You will have pain for the rest of your life. And you will never walk right again." Fortunately, I found another surgeon. I had surgery to put pins in. Ten weeks later, surgery to take the pins out. That was only the beginning. I worked with physical therapy for a few months. I was walking but still had a limp. I was determined not to fulfill the first Doctor's prophecy. After about six months of physical therapy, I noticed that I was no longer having a constant pain sensation from my foot. I worked a lot with the physical therapist, specifically on my gait, and in a few more weeks, I was walking without any noticeable hitch. After that, it was important to me to continue to walk regularly with a sense of gratitude that the simple pleasure of walking could have been taken from me.

I am a medical doctor. My specialty is not Orthopedics or Physical medicine. I have spent over 30 years helping women and couples to get pregnant. It has been an exciting journey, but it does not allow me much time to walk while working. This book will give tips for the busy person on integrating walking into your daily routine and tips for days when there is more time for a "proper" walk. This book is not meant to be a prescription. It is not medical advice. As with any exercise program, please consult your physician to ensure you are healthy for this activity level.

I have designed this book to give you tips on caring for your body while walking and with a sense of wonder and fun. Let the journey begin...

WHY WALK? WHAT IS YOUR MOTIVATION?

Walking is one of the first activities we do as children, which makes us **all** experts in walking. Walking on two legs separates us from most other animals. We walk to get ourselves from one place to another, and sometimes, we just walk.

Walking has been cherished across centuries and cultures. From the serene morning strolls of ancient Greek philosophers to the brisk urban walks in today's cities, walking remains a deeply ingrained part of human life. But beyond its historical significance, walking is a gateway to improved health, enhanced mental clarity, and a fun way to explore the world around us.

In today's world, where technology often leads to sedentary lifestyles, walking offers a natural solution to combat physical and mental health issues. The beauty of walking is its simplicity—it requires no special skills or expensive equipment and can be done almost anywhere.

Whatever your motivation is, slip on your shoes, and let's get going!

Physical Health Benefits of Walking

"A vigorous five-mile walk will do more good for an unhappy but otherwise healthy adult than all the medicine and psychology in the world." — Paul Dudley White

Cardiovascular Health

Walking has repeatedly been proven to have profound benefits for cardiovascular health. Regular walking helps reduce the risk of heart disease by lowering blood pressure, improving circulation, and strengthening the heart muscle. Studies published in the American Journal of Preventive Medicine found that walking for 30 minutes a day, five days a week, can reduce the risk of cardiovascular events by 19%. This is particularly true for individuals at risk for hypertension or those who have a family history of heart disease.

Walking increases heart rate, promoting blood circulation throughout the body. Unlike more strenuous exercises, walking remains a low-impact activity, making it accessible for people of all ages and fitness levels. Sustained, moderate exercise improves cholesterol levels by raising high-density lipoprotein (HDL) and reducing low-density lipoprotein (LDL), further contributing to heart health.

Weight Management

Walking plays a critical role in weight management. Studies have demonstrated that walking can help burn calories effectively. A person weighing 160 pounds can burn approximately 314 calories by walking briskly for an hour. Over time, regular walking can lead to significant weight loss or help maintain a healthy body weight. Walking allows for long-term sustainability, unlike high-intensity exercises, which can feel intimidating.

Moreover, walking encourages the maintenance of lean muscle mass, especially when combined with proper nutrition. This is particularly important for older adults who face age-related muscle loss.

Muscle and Bone Strengthening

Walking may not be immediately associated with muscle strengthening, but it plays a pivotal role in maintaining muscle tone and joint health. Walking strengthens muscles in the legs, hips, and abdomen, enhancing posture and balance. This is particularly valuable as we age. According to a study in the *Journal of Bone and Mineral Research*, walking helps preserve bone density, reducing the risk of osteoporosis and related fractures.

Improved Posture and Flexibility

Proper walking techniques promote better posture and alignment. Walking encourages a natural gait, which enhances core stability, reduces back pain, and improves overall flexibility. A study published in *Gait & Posture* demonstrated that consistent walking led to significant improvements in postural alignment, especially in older adults.

MENTAL AND EMOTIONAL BENEFITS

"If I could not walk far and fast, I think I should just explode and perish." —*Charles Dickens*

Stress Reduction and Mood Enhancement

Walking benefits the body and greatly enhances mental and emotional well-being. Research in the *Journal of Psychiatric Research* reveals that walking in nature, also known as "green exercise," significantly reduces stress, anxiety, and depression. Walking releases endorphins, natural chemicals in the brain that elevate mood and reduce pain.

Cognitive Health and Memory Boost

Cognitive decline is a growing concern, especially with the aging population. Walking has been linked to improved brain function and memory retention. A long-term study published in the *Journal of the American Medical Association (JAMA)* reported that older adults who walked six miles per week had a lower risk of cognitive decline compared to those with sedentary lifestyles. Walking stimulates blood flow to the brain, supporting the growth of new neural connections, thus preserving cognitive function as we age.

Walking and Sleep Quality

A well-rounded exercise routine, which includes walking, can enhance sleep quality. A study in *Sleep Medicine Reviews* highlighted that individuals who engaged in moderate exercise, such as walking, experienced fewer instances of insomnia and better overall sleep quality. This is primarily due to walking's ability to regulate circadian rhythms and reduce stress, making it easier to fall asleep and stay asleep.

Staying Active Throughout the Day

Research highlights the incredible benefits of staying active throughout the day, even in small ways. Whether taking a short walk, standing up to stretch, or simply moving more often, incorporating regular movement can be a simple and joyful way to boost your health and energy levels.

One study by **Dunstan et al.** (2012) in *Diabetes Care* shows that breaking up long periods of sitting with short walks can improve how your body manages blood sugar and insulin. It's a great reminder that even little bursts of activity can make a big difference!

Another uplifting insight from **Owen et al.** (2010) published in *circulation* emphasizes that reducing sitting time and sneaking in quick, enjoyable movement breaks throughout the day can help lower the risk of long-term health problems like heart disease and diabetes. Every step counts!

And it's not just about intense workouts — **Tremblay et al.** (2017) in *The Lancet Public Health* encourages people to weave movement into everyday life, making it fun and easy. Whether dancing around the kitchen, taking the stairs, or standing while chatting on the phone, small moments of movement can add up to big health wins.

So, stay active, keep moving, and enjoy all the feel-good benefits that come with adding more movement to your day! It's not about perfection but finding fun ways to stay engaged with your body and environment.

Choosing the Right Walking Gear: Shoes, Clothing, and Essentials

"All truly great thoughts are conceived while walking." — *Friedrich Nietzsche*

Selecting the proper walking equipment is crucial for both comfort and injury prevention. While walking may seem like a low-maintenance activity, having the right shoes, clothing, and accessories can enhance the experience, prevent blisters, and reduce the risk of musculoskeletal problems. This chapter will delve into the essentials of walking gear, from shoes to clothing, and additional tools to optimize your walking routine.

Walking Shoes: The Foundation of Comfort

Walking shoes are arguably the most essential piece of equipment for any walker. The right pair of shoes can prevent discomfort, improve performance, and protect you from injury. Research from the *Journal of Sports Science & Medicine* emphasizes that choosing appropriate footwear can significantly reduce the risk of overuse injuries like plantar fasciitis, shin splints, and tendinitis (JSSM, 2015).

Here are some key factors to consider when selecting walking shoes:

Cushioning and Support

Walking shoes should provide adequate cushioning, particularly in the heel and ball of the foot, as these areas absorb most of the impact during walking. Look for shoes with gel, foam, or air cushioning systems to reduce the stress on your joints.

Support is also critical, especially in the midsole. People with flat feet may require shoes with additional arch support, while those with high arches may benefit from shoes with more cushioning in the heel. Over time, worn-out shoes lose their supportive features, so it is essential to replace them regularly.

Flexibility and Breathability

Flexibility is essential in walking shoes, as your feet should be able to move naturally through each step. Shoes that are too stiff can restrict movement and cause discomfort. Test a shoe's flexibility by bending it at the ball of the foot. If it doesn't bend easily, it's likely too stiff for comfortable walking.

Breathable materials such as mesh or lightweight synthetics help keep your feet cool and dry, especially during long walks or in warmer weather. Shoes with moisture-wicking properties can prevent blisters caused by sweat.

Proper Fit

A well-fitted shoe is key to avoiding blisters, calluses, and other foot issues. Ensure that there's about a thumb's width of space between your longest toe and the front of the shoe to allow for natural foot expansion during walking. The heel should fit snugly to avoid slipping, and the shoe should have enough width to accommodate the natural splay of your toes.

If you have specific foot conditions such as bunions, hammertoes, or arthritis, consult with a podiatrist for custom orthotics or shoe recommendations.

Replace Shoes Regularly

Walking shoes need to be replaced periodically, depending on how much you walk and the terrain you cover. As a general guideline, most walking shoes should be replaced every 300-500 miles. It may be time for a new pair if you notice signs of wear, such as uneven tread or discomfort in your knees or feet.

Walking Clothing: Comfort, Protection, and Performance

Proper clothing can make your walk more enjoyable and efficient, especially in varying weather conditions. Your clothing should be breathable, moisture-wicking, and protect against the elements.

Moisture-Wicking Fabrics

Walking can cause you to sweat, and moisture-wicking fabrics help regulate body temperature by drawing sweat away from your skin. Look for clothes made from synthetic materials like polyester, nylon, or blends designed for active wear. These fabrics dry quickly, preventing the clammy feeling that can come with cotton when it absorbs sweat.

Brands often label these fabrics with terms like "Dri-FIT," "Clima-Cool," or "Coolmax," making it easier to identify high-performance materials.

Layering for Temperature Control

For walking in colder weather, layering is essential. Start with a moisture-wicking base layer, followed by an insulating layer such as a fleece jacket to retain body heat. Finish with a waterproof or windproof outer layer to protect against the elements. Layers can be easily adjusted as your body temperature changes during your walk.

In warmer climates, opt for lightweight, breathable fabrics that allow airflow and minimize overheating.

Sun Protection

Sun protection is crucial when walking in sunny conditions. Choose clothing with built-in UV protection or long sleeves and pants to shield your skin from the sun's rays. A wide-brimmed hat and sunglasses with UV protection can further safeguard your face and eyes.

Walking Socks: The Often-Overlooked Essential

Socks are essential in maintaining foot health during walking. Ill-fitting or poor-quality socks can cause blisters, hot spots, and discomfort.

Moisture-Wicking Socks

Like your clothing, your socks should wick away moisture to keep your feet dry. Choose socks made from synthetic fibers like polyester or merino wool, which are known for their moisture-wicking properties. Avoid cotton socks, as they tend to retain moisture, which can lead to blisters.

Padding and Seamless Design

Well-padded socks offer additional cushioning in high-impact areas like the heel and ball of the foot, helping reduce the risk of blisters and discomfort during long walks. Seamless socks are also ideal, reducing friction that could lead to chafing.

Additional Walking Accessories

While shoes and clothing are the primary walking gear, several accessories can further enhance your experience.

Walking Poles

Walking poles, often used in Nordic walking or hiking, can help improve posture, enhance cardiovascular benefits, and reduce pressure on joints, especially when walking uphill or on uneven terrain. Studies published in the *Journal of Aging and Physical Activity* indicate that walking poles may enhance stability and reduce the risk of falls in older adults.

Hydration Gear

Staying hydrated is essential during any walk, especially in warm weather or long distances. Options for hydration include handheld water bottles, hydration belts, or backpacks with built-in water reservoirs. Choose a system that allows you to drink without interrupting your walking rhythm.

Reflective Gear for Visibility

If you walk early in the morning or late in the evening, reflective gear is essential for visibility and safety. Reflective vests, armbands, or even shoes with built-in reflective strips can make you more visible to drivers and cyclists.

Tech Accessories

Wearable technology such as fitness trackers and smartwatches can help track your steps, monitor your heart rate, and provide feedback on your overall activity levels. Many fitness apps allow you to set walking goals, track routes, and even compete with friends, adding a fun, motivational aspect to your routine.

The Fun Side of Walking

"It is solved by walking." — *Saint Augustine*

You ask, "How can walking be fun?" There are many ways to make walking fun. Perhaps you are doing some of these activities already. The more you think of something as pleasurable, the more you will continue doing it.

Walking as a Social Activity

Walking can also be a social experience, offering opportunities to connect with friends, family, or strangers. Group walks or walking clubs foster a sense of community. According to a survey published in *Health Psychology*, people who walk with others are more likely to stick to their walking routines, which leads to longer-term health benefits.

Exploring Nature: Hiking and Walking Trails

Walking through nature not only provides physical benefits but also promotes mental tranquility. Hiking trails, whether through forests, mountains, or along beaches, offer a variety of experiences that stimulate the senses. Nature walks are beneficial for individuals seeking to unwind and recharge from daily stresses. Studies show that walking in natural environments enhances mental clarity and fosters creativity.

Urban Walking and Discovery

Walking is a delightful way to explore new neighborhoods, parks, and hidden gems in urban environments. It allows individuals to engage with their surroundings uniquely, encouraging spontaneous discoveries. Walking tours have become popular in many cities as people seek to combine exercise with culture and exploration.

Combining Walking with Technology

"Everywhere is within walking distance if you have the time."
— Steven Wright

Wearables and Step-Tracking: Gamifying Your Walk

Technology has transformed walking into a gamified activity. Wearable devices like Fitbits or Apple Watches allow users to track their daily steps, heart rate, and calories burned. These metrics offer real-time feedback and encouragement, making walking more engaging. A study in *The Lancet* found that individuals who use step-tracking devices are more likely to increase their daily walking activity.

Virtual Walks and VR Experiences

Virtual reality (VR) technology has also made walking an interactive experience. Platforms like Google Earth allow users to explore international destinations from the comfort of their homes. For those unable to walk outdoors due to weather or physical limitations, VR walking offers an immersive alternative.

WALKING FOR HOLISTIC WELLNESS

"I only went out for a walk, and finally concluded to stay out till sundown, for going out,I found, was really going in."
—John Muir

Walking is not only a physical exercise but can also be a practice that nurtures holistic wellness. When combined with mindfulness, meditation, and spiritual practices, walking becomes a pathway to mental clarity and emotional well-being. Many ancient traditions emphasize walking as a form of meditation or spiritual journey, from Buddhist walking meditation to Christian pilgrimages.

Mindful Walking

Mindful walking involves focusing on the sensations of each step, the movement of the body, and the surrounding environment, fostering a deep connection between the mind and body. Studies from the *Journal of Behavioral Medicine* suggest that mindful walking can reduce symptoms of anxiety, depression, and stress.

How to Practice Mindful Walking

- Walk at a slow, steady pace, paying close attention to each step.

- Focus on your breath and the movement of your body. Feel the sensation of your feet connecting with the ground.

- Allow thoughts to come and go without judgment, focusing on the present moment.

- Use your senses to observe your environment—listen to the sounds, notice the colors, and feel the air on your skin.

Walking as Meditation

Walking meditation is a traditional practice that blends physical movement with meditation techniques. This practice, common in Buddhism, helps cultivate mindfulness and present-moment awareness. Walking slowly with intention while breathing deeply brings both mental relaxation and physical calmness.

Spiritual Walking Traditions

- **Pilgrimages**: Walking pilgrimages, such as the Camino de Santiago in Spain, are spiritual journeys undertaken to enhance personal reflection and growth.

- **Labyrinth Walking**: Walking a labyrinth is an ancient spiritual practice used for meditation and prayer, often in a slow, reflective manner. This practice can help individuals center themselves and find peace during stressful times.

WALKING FOR SPECIAL POPULATIONS

"An early-morning walk is a blessing for the whole day." — *Henry David Thoreau*

Walking is one of the most adaptable forms of exercise and can be tailored to the needs of various populations. Whether it's pregnant women, older adults, children, or those with specific health conditions, walking provides accessible physical activity for nearly everyone. Understanding how to modify walking routines for special populations is essential for safety and effectiveness.

Walking During Pregnancy

Walking is a recommended form of exercise for pregnant women due to its low-impact nature and cardiovascular benefits. The *American*

College of Obstetricians and Gynecologists (ACOG) suggests that pregnant women engage in moderate physical activity, like walking for 150 minutes per week, which can help manage weight gain, reduce pregnancy-related discomfort, and promote mental well-being.

Benefits of Walking for Pregnant Women

- **Improved Circulation**: Walking helps prevent blood clots and varicose veins, which are common during pregnancy.

- **Reduction of Back Pain**: Gentle walking strengthens muscles in the lower back and abdomen, alleviating pregnancy-related back pain.

- **Mood Enhancement**: Walking releases endorphins, which help manage the emotional fluctuations often experienced during pregnancy.

Tips for Safe Walking During Pregnancy

- Wear supportive shoes and maternity support belts if needed.

- Avoid uneven or slippery surfaces to prevent falls.

- Stay hydrated and avoid walking during the hottest parts of the day.

- Consult a healthcare provider, especially if experiencing complications like high blood pressure or gestational diabetes.

Walking for Older Adults

As we age, maintaining physical activity is vital for preventing age-related conditions such as osteoporosis, arthritis, and cardiovascular disease. Walking offers a low-risk exercise that promotes mobility, reduces the risk of falls, and enhances cognitive function. A study in the *Journal of the American Geriatrics Society* showed that regular walking reduced fall risk by improving balance and coordination in older adults.

Benefits for Seniors

- **Bone Health**: Weight-bearing exercises like walking help maintain bone density and reduce the risk of fractures.

- **Improved Cognitive Function**: Walking boosts blood flow to the brain, which helps slow cognitive decline.

- **Joint Mobility**: Gentle walking can alleviate stiffness associated with arthritis, promoting better joint health and flexibility.

Walking Tips for Older Adults

- Use walking poles or canes for added stability if needed.

- Choose safe, flat surfaces with clear walking paths.

- Wear well-fitting shoes with good arch support and cushioning to prevent joint strain.

- Walk with a buddy or group for added safety and social interaction.

Walking with Children: Fun and Educational

Walking with children offers an excellent opportunity for physical activity while promoting curiosity and discovery. Encouraging children to walk regularly can help establish healthy habits early in life. Research published in the *International Journal of Behavioral Nutrition and Physical Activity* indicates that children who engage in regular walking or physical activity are less likely to develop obesity and have better academic performance.

Fun Walking Ideas for Families

- **Scavenger Hunts**: Create a list of items for children to find while walking, such as different types of leaves, birds, or street signs.

- **Story Walks**: Make up a story while walking, allowing children to contribute to the plot as they encounter various objects and people along the way.

- **Nature Walks**: Children can learn about their environment by walking through nature reserves, parks, or even urban spaces while observing plants, animals, and ecosystems.

Tips for Walking with Children

- Keep walks short and engaging to match their attention span.

- Allow for frequent breaks, and bring water and snacks.

- Choose safe routes that avoid heavy traffic.

WALKING SAFETY TIPS

"Walking is the best possible exercise. Habituate yourself to walk very far." —Thomas Jefferson

Staying safe while walking is crucial, particularly in environments with potential hazards such as traffic, uneven terrain, or harsh weather conditions. Taking the necessary precautions can help prevent injuries, allowing you to walk comfortably and confidently.

Proper Footwear and Clothing

As covered earlier, the right shoes and clothing are essential for walking safety. Well-fitting shoes can prevent blisters and foot pain, while moisture-wicking clothing keeps the body cool and dry.

Walking on Safe Paths

Use sidewalks, pedestrian pathways, or designated walking lanes to avoid traffic when walking in urban areas. In rural or natural areas, stay on marked trails to reduce the risk of getting lost or encountering hazardous terrain. Wear reflective gear or carry a flashlight when walking in low-visibility conditions (e.g., at dusk or dawn).

Hydration and Nutrition

Proper hydration is critical during walks, especially in hot weather. Drink water before, during, and after walking, even if you don't feel thirsty. On longer walks, especially hikes, pack portable snacks such as nuts, energy bars, or fruit to maintain your energy levels.

Stay Aware of Your Surroundings

Distractions such as listening to loud music or using your phone can prevent you from noticing hazards like approaching cars, bicycles, or uneven ground. While listening to music or podcasts is okay, keep the volume low enough to remain aware of your surroundings.

Medical Considerations

For individuals with pre-existing medical conditions, such as heart disease or diabetes, consult a healthcare professional before beginning any new walking regimen. Carry any necessary medications, like inhalers or glucose tablets, if you have conditions that may require immediate attention during a walk.

Conclusion: Walking Your Way to a Happier, Healthier Life

Walking is far more than a simple mode of transportation—it's a lifestyle that combines physical, mental, emotional, and even spiritual wellness. Whether you're a beginner taking your first walks or an experienced walker looking for new ways to enhance your routine, walking offers an accessible and enjoyable way to improve your health.

You can turn this humble activity into a lifelong journey toward better health and greater happiness by focusing on proper technique, selecting the right gear, and tailoring walks to your specific needs and goals. Walking is therapeutic and refreshing, offering a way to unwind, reflect, and discover the world around you. So step out, explore, and walk your way to a better you.

If you liked this book or found some good information to help you put some fun into your walk routine, I would appreciate a review on Amazon.com. If you have some ways that help you enjoy walking please put them in a review. I might include them in the next edition of this book!

Ten Ways to Put Some Fun in Your Walk

1. Smile when you are walking. Smile at people walking by. Greet them with "Good morning" or the appropriate time of day. If they are walking a pet, greet the pet too. Having a smile on your face will automatically make the walk more fun.

2. Look at the world around you. Pick out something you haven't seen before (i.e., a flower, sunlight streaming through the trees, a sign in the window, the color of a house or building). Say some words of gratitude for that item.

3. Pick a different route. If you do the same route every day, it can become tiresome. If you usually go right, try starting to the left. Explore different neighborhoods close to your home

or drive to a park and walk.

4. Make short goals within your longer walk. Use your pedometer or stopwatch. Choose a short distance - the next 3 mailboxes or to the next corner. Go full out for that distance and see how fast you can go. Keep track to see how you improve, or choose different segments to make your fast run.

5. Have a ball while you walk. Use a basketball or tennis ball and bounce it as you walk. You can also buy a ball on a cord so it will always come back to you. Using a ball has the added advantage of increasing upper body strength and coordination.

6. Listen to music or podcasts while you walk. Music can help you with a beat to pace yourself. Podcasts can help you keep up with information, but try something lighter that will elevate your mood. Many comedy show podcasts can keep you laughing while you walk.

7. Interact with nature. Listen for the sounds of nature while you are walking - the rustling of the trees to a breeze. The movement of leaves or how the sunlight plays along. The blueness of the sky and how the clouds are moving. The smell of freshly cut grass. The feel of the road beneath your feet. If you keep a journal, log your experience when you

return home.

8. If you are walking on a sidewalk, you can play games on the cracks. As children, we used to play a game to avoid the cracks. You must change your gait to avoid the cracks, making you watch your steps more carefully. Or switch it up and step on all the cracks.

9. Pick a color of the day. If you are on a street with a good amount of traffic, count the number of cars you see in that color. See what color is the most common in your area.

10. Walk with another person. Besides giving motivation for walking, just being with another person can lift your spirits. The nice thing about walking over running is that you are going at a pace that allows conversation. Discuss with your partner that you are going to talk about positive things or talk about things in a positive way. Even when discussing a problem, if you talk about some of the good things that came out of it, your mind will be focused more on the possibilities of the solution than on just the problem.